IIIII II IIIIIIIII IIIIIIIIIII III III
I0101809

Dr. Guide Book Series

PREVENTING ASTHMA ATTACKS

By Kenneth Wright
In consultation with the National Institute of Health and
National Heart, Lung and Blood Institute, Allergy, Asthma
Information Association (AAIA), Physicians Association for
Patient Education and the American Academy of Allergy,
Asthma and Immunology (AAAAI).

The publisher Mediscript Communications Inc.
acknowledges the financial support of the Government of
Canada through the Book Publishing Industry Development
Program (BPIDP) for our publishing activities.

Distributed by MACLEAN Communications Inc.
Tel: (905) 849 9752
Email: Kathy@macleancomm.com

ISBN 978-1-896616-01-8

TABLE OF CONTENTS

INTRODUCTION

You may be reading this book because you or a family member (often a child) has asthma and you want to take control and enjoy a normal life and experience no dangerous "asthma attacks".

Conversely a great many people do not know they have asthma and you may want to find out more about this health condition for yourself or a child. There are in fact a whole array of ambiguous symptoms from breathlessness, wheezing, chest tightness, coughing to cold symptoms that may or may not be asthma. Each person's asthma condition is unique in both the symptoms and causes.

Your medical team often considers this book as important as the asthma medication because how you help yourself or a loved one with asthma is a very important part of the treatment. This book can provide basic understanding and help you or a family member effectively manage this condition.

The medication available for asthma patients can be remarkably effective and only a general explanation is provided on the types of medication available within this book. This is the domain of the physician / asthma educator and explanations, training with written or other material should be provided by the medical team

Perhaps one of the most important aspects of this book, aside from gaining understanding of asthma, is how you can actually prevent an asthma attack by avoiding the causes (called triggers).

In conclusion this book can:
Help you understand the basics of asthma
Provide tips on how to avoid the causes (triggers) of asthma
Help you monitor and control of your asthma.

Finally and most importantly, the result of the last three points can assist you in avoiding a dangerous asthma attack which may involve

UNDERSTANDING ASTHMA

Here's a selection of asthma patients' comments about their symptoms:

Glenda Brooking, 62:
"It felt like a pressure on my chest – a very uncomfortable feeling."

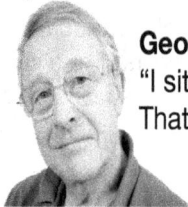

George Taylor, 73:
"I sit up at night – I just can't get my breath. That's what scared me."

Jane Wilson, 15:
"It's like a Mack truck sitting on your chest."

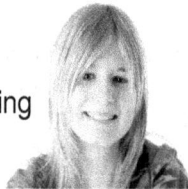

Cameron Blair, 14
"It's hard to get your breath – just short fast breaths instead of usual deep breaths."

It is estimated that there are 22 million people diagnosed with asthma in North America; nearly nine million of them are children.

More than 5000 North Americans will die from an asthma attack this year. It is believed a large percentage of those deaths could be prevented through understanding and preventative actions.

WHO IS AT RISK

☞ Asthma is common, affecting 5 – 10% of the population.

☞ Asthma is one of the most common conditions of childhood.

☞ Asthma is closely linked to allergies.

☞ Asthma can run in families.

☞ Most but not all people with asthma have allergies.

☞ Children with a family history of allergy and asthma are more likely to have asthma.

☞ Although asthma affects people of all ages, it most often starts in childhood.

☞ More boys have asthma than girls.

☞ In adulthood, more women have asthma than men.

☞ Although asthma affects people of all races, African American are more likely than Caucasians to be hospitalized for asthma attacks.

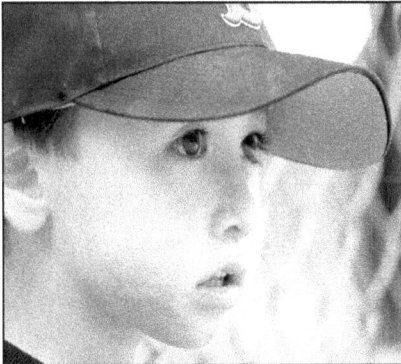

DO YOU HAVE ASTHMA?

	YES	NO
I wheeze (breathing out with a noisy whistling sound)	☐	☐
I cough due to stuff (mucus) in my airways which:		
Makes it hard to sleep at night	☐	☐
Is often worse at night	☐	☐
Is often worse in the morning	☐	☐
I have a tight feeling in my chest like something sitting on it or squeezing it	☐	☐
I have shortness of breath–just can't get enough air	☐	☐
I often gasp–trying to get more air inside me	☐	☐
I have trouble talking due to air intake	☐	☐
I have difficulty walking or doing things because of lack of air	☐	☐
I have faster breathing or noisy breathing	☐	☐
I spit up phlegm (mucus)	☐	☐
The symptom(s) listed above are variable and reversible with me	☐	☐

If you answered Yes to any of these symptoms you should be checked by your physician for asthma. If you answered Yes to most of these questions there is a strong chance you have asthma.

WHAT ASTHMA FEELS LIKE
We will try to demonstrate and explain
what asthma feels like.

First, make a tight fist and press it firmly to your lips. Then try to breathe in and then out through your mouth. You should find it very difficult to breathe. That is exactly what asthma is like.

Another way to describe it is to breathe through a straw–you should be able to breathe easily. Think of the straw as one of the airways to your lungs. Now pinch the straw, so that it becomes narrower. Try breathing in and out through the pinched straw. You will find breathing again much harder – that, too is what asthma is like.

Everybody's asthma is unique; some people may have annual asthma attacks (sometimes called episodes) each year, when they have real difficulty breathing and have to go to Emergency. For others, who never have an attack, asthma is merely an inconvenience.

Up to 10% of North Americans will suffer from asthma symptoms in their lifetime. For some, it can be a chronic respiratory condition, an issue they have to deal with most of their lives. On the other hand, children with asthma often lose their symptoms as they grow older.

In spite of the number of sufferers, the increasing numbers of new cases and the constant threat of attacks, asthma is still one of the most misunderstood health issues of the day. False claims about asthma abound: people believe it's contagious, or is caused by anxiety, bad parenting, etc. This book dispels these myths and provides you with a positive, controlling outlook on this condition.

GOOD NEWS ABOUT ASTHMA

Unlike other respiratory diseases like bronchitis and emphysema, asthma does not tend to cause permanent damage.

There are excellent prescription medications available from your physician and pharmacist to treat asthma either by relieving symptoms (reliever medications) or by controlling them on a long term basis and preventing attacks (preventer medications).

You can learn to monitor and predict asthma attacks or prevent them altogether.

You can find out what there is in the environment or in your lifestyle that might bring on or trigger an asthma attack or symptoms and take measures to minimize it.

Asthma is not contagious; you cannot pass it on to someone else like the flu or a cold.

Understanding this health condition and working with your physician on a treatment and prevention plan will give you the power to take part in your own treatment and enjoy a healthy, active life without fear of disability or being hospitalized.

The bottom line is that what you thought was a frightening condition can become nothing more than an occasional inconvenience. All the good news above will become more meaningful as you continue reading this book.

HOW ASTHMA WORKS

Asthma is a chronic disease that affects your breathing passages. People who do not have asthma are able to move air freely in and out of the lungs.

With asthma, air cannot pass freely in and out of the lungs because these airways are sensitive or "twitchy".

Have you ever walked into a room that has just been painted? Do you remember the strong smell? A person with asthma can have an asthma attack due to this irritant. A room full of cigarette smoke can have the same effect.

To explain this more fully, we know we breathe through our mouths and air goes through airways to our lungs. When you have asthma the airways go a little smaller. The main reason for this is due to inflammation; this is the same reaction when you are bitten by a mosquito or receive a bad scratch or burn on your skin. These all cause redness and swelling, which is what happens to your airways when you have asthma.

As well as inflammation of the airways, two other factors contribute to asthma:

1.The muscles around the airways go into spasm and tighten, further narrowing the airways.

2.Glands in the airways secrete more mucus, caused by this inflammation, making you cough.

PROCESS OF ASTHMA

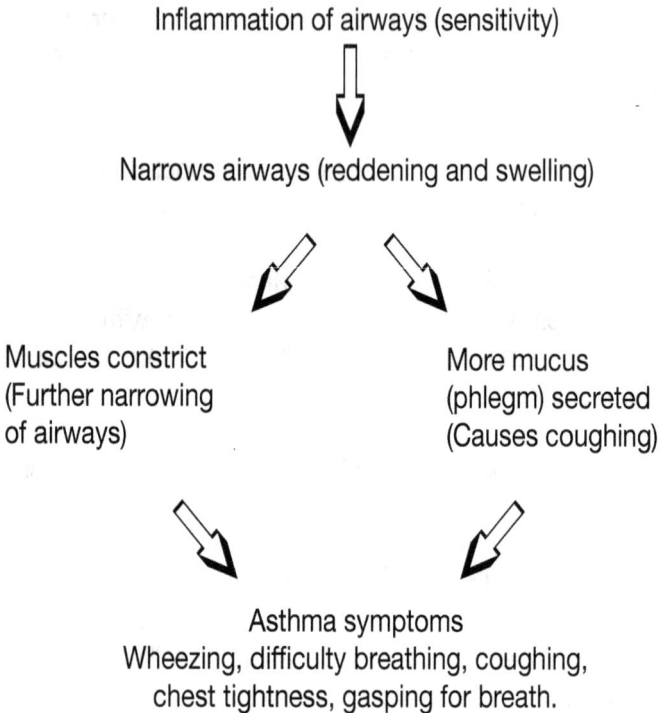

Inflammation of airways (sensitivity)

⬇

Narrows airways (reddening and swelling)

Muscles constrict
(Further narrowing
of airways)

More mucus
(phlegm) secreted
(Causes coughing)

Asthma symptoms
Wheezing, difficulty breathing, coughing,
chest tightness, gasping for breath.

Asthma is a fairly complex health condition but as you can see from the above flow chart, the fundamental causative factor seems to be inflammation of the airways to the lungs. As we put it another way earlier, asthma sufferers have sensitive or "**twitchy**" airways.

You will learn later on that one of the key approaches to treatment is to reduce or eliminate this inflamation in the airways through medication. A symbolic way of understanding the role of inflammation of the airways is to look at the following chart which shows how symptoms become more severe as inflammation increases:

HIGHEST

10	Serious asthma attack perhaps
9	requiring hospitalization.

8	Asthma attack requiring emergency
7	reliever medication.

6	Asthma symptoms requiring purposeful treatment to prevent symptoms worsening; perhaps gasping for breath.

Inflamation of the airways

5	Difficulty breathing, some shortness of breath during the night, runny nose.

4	Mild cough with some phlegm that goes
3	away after a week.

2	After having a cold you continue to have a cough for a couple of weeks.

1	Slight wheezing after exercising or a stressful event in your life.

LOWEST

0	Breathing normally, no symptoms at all.

THE ABC OF PREVENTING ASTHMA ATTACKS

The following are the 3 primary methods you can take to prevent asthma attacks:

Avoid the triggers that cause your asthma attacks. This is the most natural and common sense approach to preventing symptoms or an attack.

Be prepared: know your treatment plan, including emergency procedures and how and when to use your medications.

Control the progress of your asthma through knowing the warning signs and using a peak flow meter.

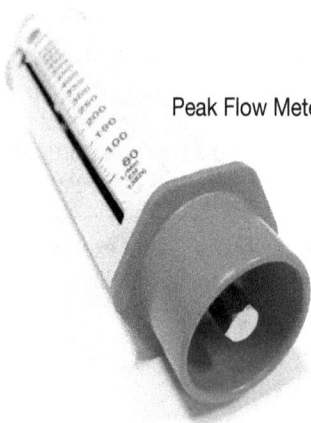

Peak Flow Meter

TESTING FOR ASTHMA

There are a variety of simple asthma tests:

1. Your history of symptoms.

Initially, your physician has to be like a detective and ask you questions about your symptoms and level of discomfort. He or she will also be looking for clues as to what may have brought on the asthma–was it after exercise, exposure to cigarette smoke, allergies? If you have a chance before going to the physician, try to fill out the diary in this book. You can often forget symptoms after a few days whereas documenting your symptoms over time can help your physician to correctly diagnose your condition.

2. Peak flow rate assessment.

A simple but quantifiable way of determining the extent of your asthma is the peak flow meter test. It is easy to use and many asthmatics use the meter at home to monitor how they are managing their asthma.

Your physician, technician or nurse will ask you to blow as hard and as fast as you can through the meter. (The best analogy to this would be blowing out the candles at your birthday party.) Just as scales measure your weight and a thermometer measures your temperature, this peak flow meter measures the maximum speed with which air can be forced out of your lungs.

If your airways are narrowed due to inflammation, then you will not be able to achieve as great a speed as normal and therefore you will have a reduced peak flow rate.

For example, if the patient is a 5'1", 12-year-old boy, one would expect a normal reading of around 361. The peak flow rate, however, is measuring just 240, considerably below the average for his age, height and gender. This indicates he has narrowing of his airways and may have asthma.

Further to this test the physician may want you to exercise on a bike or treadmill or give you some medication to also assess your lung efficiency changes.

3. Pulmonary function test.

"Pulmonary" is a term that refers to the lungs. Someone from your medical team will ask you to breathe while you are hooked up to tubes and equipment that measures how your lungs are performing.

Other tests that may be done to determine any other causes other than asthma are chest x-rays and laboratory tests on the mucus you are coughing up.

Allergy Tests

Because asthma is often triggered by allergies, you may be given tests whereby a drop of a possible allergen trigger like dust, pollen or mold is placed in rows on the arm. Each drop is then gently pricked to see if there is a reaction. This is very safe and the skin reaction settles down after 30 - 60 minutes.

Alternatively, instead of testing your skin reaction to allergens you can have a blood test where a laboratory computer can analyze, from chemicals in your blood, what types of allergens trigger your asthma attacks.

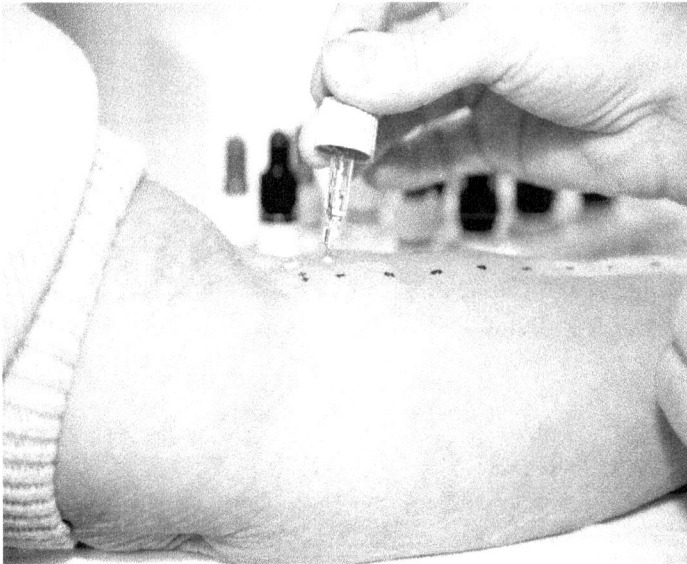

FIRST VISIT TO THE PHYSICIAN

Rose Perry, 44, is a business executive with 2 teenage children. She lives in the country, a 30-minute commute by train from her office downtown. Until now her only health problem was an allergy to her cats, which she eventually had to give away to a family member, and a broken ankle 10 years ago when skiing.

Doctor:
Hello Rose, we had our yearly check-up 6 months ago. What brings you in today?

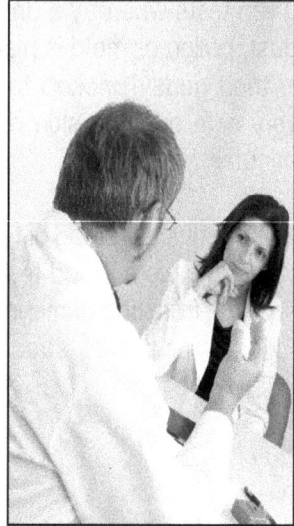

Rose Perry:
Well, I seem to have a few problems that make me concerned about my heart. When I go for long walks I start to get a tightness in my chest after about half an hour. So I stop and rest for a bit but it doesn't go away. And lately I seem to get tired more quickly than I used to–I feel like I can't get my breath.

Doctor:
That tightness in your chest–do you ever get it at any other time?

Rose:
Actually, I do. I get it when I'm stressed about meeting deadlines at work.

Doctor:
Now on your last check-up, your heart seemed very healthy. You'll remember I had you do an EEG and you seemed very fit. Have you had any pins and needles feeling in your hands or palpitations in your heart?

Rose:
No, nothing like that.

Doctor:
How about colds, flu, coughs, runny nose–anything like that over the last few months?

Rose:
Just the normal things I suppose. I have had a few colds and every now and then I get a cough that lasts for a while. I bring up phlegm, but I take Neo Citran and that seems to help.

Doctor:
Can you ever remember making a sort of whistling noise when you breathe out, a wheezing that comes from deep within your chest?

Rose:
Why yes, sometimes when I'm concentrating on a stressful project at work, I'll get that chest tightness, and then for a while after I try to compose myself, there's a funny sound that I can't do anything about–I suppose it could be like a whistle.

Doctor:
Remember the symptoms you had when you had your cats–the runny nose, watery eyes, the sneezing. Have you ever had anything like that during the last few months?

Rose:
Oh, no, nothing like those symptoms from the cats – they used to sleep on the bed–I would start sneezing and it would just go on and on. It was unbearable. No, I haven't had anything that intense. But I do have these occasional sneezing periods now and then–just 2 or 3 sneezes at a time and then a cough seem to develop from it–nothing serious, just an irritation.

Doctor:
Can you remember your last sneezing bout? Was it in the morning? Do you remember what you were doing?

Rose:
Actually, I was in bed. John always jokes that I must be allergic to him, because I often have those sneezing episodes when I get into bed.

Doctor:
I think I know what your problem is. I'm going to check your heart in a minute, but I would like you first to blow into this peak flow meter. Blow as hard and as fast as you can until you can't blow any more.

Rose blows into the peak flow meter.

Doctor:
Well, this tells us a story, Rose. We'll have to do a few more tests but it looks like you have adult onset asthma. This can be managed quite easily with medication and your cooperation.

Rose:
Asthma? But I'm in my forties–I thought it was mostly kids that had asthma?

Doctor:
It's actually quite common for adults to develop asthma. There's a link between allergies and asthma and I suspect that because you have had a predisposition to allergies, through your cats, you may well have developed a sensitivity to another allergen. And I'm thinking that since you tend to sneeze when you get into bed you may have developed an allergy to the dust mites that often live in mattresses. There's a lot of clinical evidence out there confirming that dust mites can trigger asthma attacks. I'd like you to be tested by an allergist to check if you have dust mite or other allergies.

Rose:
But what actually causes asthma?

Doctor:
For unknown reasons people with asthma have unusually sensitive airways, the tubes or bronchi that carry air to the lungs. Asthma results from an inflammation in the tissue that lines these airways, inflammation not unlike the swelling and redness you get when you are bitten by a mosquito in your garden. Coupled with this inflammation, your airways can become narrower and the phlegm or mucus produced inside them causes you to cough. This makes breathing even more difficult.

Rose:
Is it life-threatening? Should I be worried?

Doctor:
People can die of asthma attacks but it's not common. You're fortunate because you don't seem have developed a serious asthma attack where you're gasping for breath. It seems the good news for you is that you get plenty of warning and the symptoms are just inconvenient and mild.

You'll have to familiarize yourself with this condition and after you've been tested for allergies we'll prepare a treatment plan for you. I'll have our nurse explain to you how to use a peak flow meter so that you can measure how well you are breathing.

Rose:
In some ways I'm glad I have asthma–I came to you because I thought my heart was the problem.

Doctor:
You know, the sad fact is that there are thousands of people who have asthma and don't know it–they think the problem is with their heart. And then there are others who think it's just a harmless allergy to something, or a cold or bronchitis.

Conclusion
Rose was diagnosed with asthma and tests by her allergist confirmed she was allergic to cats, dust mites and house dust. She was prescribed two medications, a preventer medication which she takes twice a day and she also has a reliever medicine (a puffer) which she inhales when she experiences asthma symptoms. She thinks the asthma is brought on mostly by stress, cold weather or the occasional time she is exposed to cats at the home of a relative. Rose lives a relatively normal life and has never had to go to Emergency due to an asthma attack.

THE ASTHMA QUIZ

	TRUE	FALSE
1. Asthma is a common disease among children and adults.	☐	☐
2. Asthma is an emotional or psychological illness.	☐	☐
3. The way parents raise children can cause asthma.	☐	☐
4. Asthma attacks or episodes may cause breathing problems but they are not really harmful or dangerous.	☐	☐
5. Asthma attacks usually occur without warning.	☐	☐
6. Many different things can bring on an asthma attack.	☐	☐
7. Asthma cannot be cured but it can be controlled.	☐	☐
8. Both children and adults can have asthma.	☐	☐
9. Tobacco smoke can bring on an asthma attack.	☐	☐
10. People with asthma should not exercise.	☐	☐

Next page **ANSWERS**

1. TRUE. Asthma is a common disease among children and adults and it is increasing. In North America 20 million people have asthma, of whom 5 million are under 18 years of age.

2. FALSE. Asthma is not an emotional or psychological disease, although strong emotions can make asthma worse. People with asthma have sensitive airways to the lungs that can react to certain things, causing the airways to tighten and fill with mucus. These people then have trouble breathing.

3. FALSE. The way parents raise their children does not bring on asthma. It is not caused by being overprotective or an unhappy relationship between the parent and child.

4. FALSE. Asthma attacks can be very harmful. People can be hospitalized and some have even died from an asthma attack. That is why it is important to know how to control or prevent the asthma attack.

5. FALSE. Sometimes an asthma attack can come on quickly. However, before a person has any wheezing or shortness of breath there are usually warning signs such as a cough, a scratchy throat or tightness in the chest. You can learn to recognize these early warning signs and take medicine to prevent an attack.

6. TRUE. An asthma attack can be brought on by many different things–or triggers as they're called. Each person with asthma has an individual set of "asthma triggers"–it could be pollen for one person or the irritation of paint fumes for someone else.

7. TRUE. There is no cure yet for asthma. The good news is that asthma can be controlled through common sense, medications and understanding.

8. TRUE. Both children and adults can have asthma. Sometimes, symptoms such as shortness of breath will go away as the child becomes older. And sometimes the symptoms of asthma are not recognized until a child is an adult.

9. TRUE. Smoke from cigarettes, pipes or cigars can bring on asthma symptoms and an attack. Indoor smoky air from fireplaces and outdoor smog can make asthma worse. The best plan is not to smoke.

10. FALSE. Exercise is beneficial for most of us, whether we have asthma or not. A person with his or her asthma under control can play most sports, and warming up exercises or medicines taken before exercising can prevent asthma symptoms. A number of Olympic gold medalists have asthma.

KNOW YOUR WARNING SIGNS

It is rare for an asthma attack to come on suddenly without warning. It's your responsibility to know your warning signs so that you can take action and prevent the symptoms from becoming worse.

Here is a list of common early warning signs. Make a note of the ones you've experienced and add any other warning signs not on the list:

- Waking up at least two nights in a row due to coughing, wheezing or shortness of breath
- Decreased effect or increased usage of your reliever medication
- Early morning wheezing
- Tightness of your chest
- Asthma symptoms affecting your daily activities
- Shortness of breath
- Faster breathing
- Itchy or sore throat
- Dark circles under the eyes
- Other warning signs you experience:

....

....

....

THE CAUSES (TRIGGERS) OF ASTHMA

We have learnt that in simple terms the underlying common reason for asthma is inflamed or sensitive airways – or in slang terms, "twitchy" airways.

The extent of the inflammation brings on symptoms such as shortness of breath, wheezing, coughing, chest tightness and so on.

The $64,000 question is "what causes these symptoms". Sadly there is no universal answer, each person has his or her sensitivity to the causes or triggers. However for the patient, by finding out these causes or triggers and then with some thoughtful analysis, you can prevent asthma attacks and enjoy a normal life.

So what are these triggers or causes. The answer is in your environment, your home and the outside. There are known airborne particles that can not only be=ring on allergy attacks but can also trigger asthma attacks or symptoms.

These triggers include cat and dog dander, house dust, mites, pollen, air pollution, sprays, fumes, tobacco smoke, molds, cockroaches and more. The good news is that you can avoid these triggers to some degree, especially in the home. The outside triggers are more difficult to avoid but you can take steps to minimize exposure.

The following section overviews these triggers and provides tips to avoid exposure.

ASTHMA TRIGGERS IN THE HOME

The following general tips can provide overall improvement of your home environment.

Home environment control checklist::

☞ Complete your bedroom checklist and focus on improving this room (see next section).

☞ Install air purifier(s) appropriate for your needs.

☞ Have your furnace professionally inspected.

☞ Ensure your air ducts are regularly professionally cleaned.

☞ Use effective vacuum cleaners–either central vacuum systems or HEPA vacuums.

☞ Install a hygrometer to check your humidity.

☞ Keep your relative humidity below 50%.

☞ Remove or minimize carpets throughout the house. Replace old carpets.

☞ Avoid clutter–this promotes dust-catching.

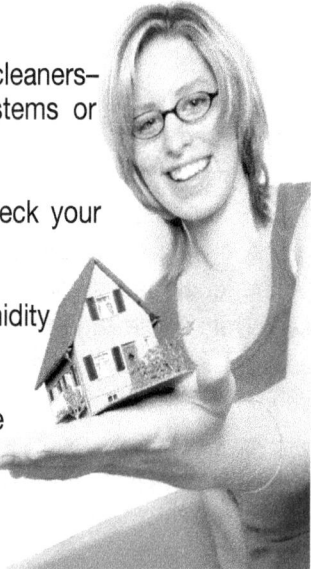

THE BEDROOM

You probably spend about a third of your life in the bedroom. It follows, then, that you breathe the air in your bedroom about a third of your life.

If you can clear allergens and irritants from this area, your respiratory system (nose, throat, airways, and lungs) can build up strength and resistance to the barrage of allergens and irritants in areas that are harder to control.

Once you accept that the bedroom should be the focus of your efforts, look at the following guidelines:

☞ Eliminate upholstered chairs, rugs, drapes, and leather furniture.

☞ Floors should be wood or linoleum.

☞ Furniture should be made of wood, plastic, or metal.

☞ Position the bed away from air vents; do not store anything underneath it.

☞ Virtually everything should be washable, including the bedding.

☞ Do not allow pets in the bedroom.

☞ Keep closets neat. Do not store blankets, woolens, sports equipment, and hats in the bedroom closet.

☞ Store clothing in zippered bags.

☞ Use synthetic pillows, preferably dacron or foam. Do not use feather, down, or kapok. Wash pillows monthly. Quilts and sleeping bags also should contain synthetic filling.

☞ Avoid dust-catchers and cluttered surfaces. Keep books, ornaments, and mobiles to a minimum.

☞ If there are vents in the room, cover them with cheese cloth or another appropriate material. If you have baseboard heating, remove the front and sides, so that you can vacuum inside. Dust is a major irritant.

☞ Doors and windows should fit tightly and should be kept closed during pollen and pollution alerts. Keep the windows clean, inside and out.

☞ Clean the room at least twice a week with a damp mop and a damp dust cloth.

☞ Vacuum mattresses frequently and encase them and the pillows in allergy-proof covers with zippers. Replace mattresses every ten years.

☞ Keep children's toys in a box with a lid.

☞ Use synthetic blankets.

☞ Do not use venetian blinds or long drapes. Curtains or shades should be made of a smooth, washable cotton or synthetic. Roll-up shades are preferable.

☞ Installing an air-conditioner can substantially improve air quality.

☞ Keep the decor simple, with as few accessories (including artwork) as possible.

☞ If additional heat is needed, use an electric heater.

☞ Do not use flowers, perfumes, powders, or scented candles.

☞ The walls and ceiling should be washable.

☞ Make it an iron-clad rule that clutter be dramatically reduced or eliminated.

Remember, you and your family probably spend about eight hours a day in the bedroom. The purer the air, the less challenge to the respiratory system and the greater the probability of reduced allergy symptoms. Tick off the items on the checklist as you achieve them. Thoroughness is the key!

Bedroom Cleaning and Maintenance Guidelines

	Week							
	1	2	3	4	5	6	7	8
Tidy up clutter.	☐	☐	☐	☐	☐	☐	☐	☐
Do not use brooms or dry dusters.	☐	☐	☐	☐	☐	☐	☐	☐
Use water, not sprays, as a cleaner.	☐	☐	☐	☐	☐	☐	☐	☐
Wash walls and ceiling periodically.	☐	☐	☐	☐	☐	☐	☐	☐
Damp mop and dust twice a week.	☐	☐	☐	☐	☐	☐	☐	☐
Clean the windows.	☐	☐	☐	☐	☐	☐	☐	☐
Vacuum nonwashable items.	☐	☐	☐	☐	☐	☐	☐	☐
Vacuum mattress and box spring each time linens are changed.	☐	☐	☐	☐	☐	☐	☐	☐
Wipe mattress covers weekly.	☐	☐	☐	☐	☐	☐	☐	☐
Vacuum carpet at least once a week.	☐	☐	☐	☐	☐	☐	☐	☐
Empty vacuum outside the room. Keep door closed.	☐	☐	☐	☐	☐	☐	☐	☐
If sensitive, wear a face mask.	☐	☐	☐	☐	☐	☐	☐	☐

COCKROACHES

It is estimated that 40% of asthma sufferers are sensitive to cockroaches. Again, like dust mites, their bodily waste can trigger asthma or allergy symptoms.

Cockroaches are attracted to food and to warm, moist areas such as:

- Kitchen cabinets
- Damp basements
- Upholstered furniture
- Soft furnishings
- Bedrooms

- Kitchen floors
- Mattresses
- Bathrooms
- Toilets

PREVENTATIVE MEASURES

☞ Reduce food sources:

☞ Restrict all eating to the dining room and kitchen. Use trays if eating elsewhere.

☞ Wash dirty dishes and counters immediately.

☞ Clean up crumbs and spills immediately.

☞ Ensure food garbage is tightly sealed in one garbage can which is emptied and cleaned often.

☞ Don't leave your pet's food out overnight.

☞ Store all dry foods in sealed containers.

☞ Clean drawers regularly. Dispose of junk.

☞ Throw away or recycle paper products (especially from the grocery store).

☞ Reduce dampness.

☞ Remove rotted flooring and damp wallpaper.
Fix leaking pipes.

☞ Waterproof cement floors in the garage and basement. Cover with plastic to prevent moisture from rising.

☞ Repair cracks in the foundation.

☞ Install a dehumidifier.

Also, close entry points with a sealant and talk to your local hardware store for advice.
If a cockroach infestation is severe, consider using a professional exterminator.

INDOOR AIR POLLUTION

North Americans can spend as much as 90% of their time indoors; aside from the common triggers already mentioned there can be numerous fumes and airborne chemicals within the home that can trigger asthma symptoms. For example, if you have paints or other volatile products in your house, either get rid of them or seal them and put them in a shed or in the garage.

PREVENTATIVE MEASURES

Options include avoidance, elimination, sealing or placing the pollutant in an isolated area. Improving ventilation can also help. Anything with a strong odor, like aerosols, new carpets or paint sprays, can trigger an asthma attack in some people.

Here is a list of possible asthma triggers for you to check:

☐ Car exhaust
☐ Kerosene
☐ Ammonia
☐ Perfumes
☐ Dry cleaning fluid
☐ Swimming pool
☐ Bleaches
☐ Paint
☐ Marking pens
☐ Natural gas
☐ Motor oil
☐ Disinfectants
☐ Aerosol sprays
☐ Solvents
☐ Strong odors

☐ Furnace
☐ Glue
☐ Floor waxes
☐ Tobacco
☐ Moth balls
☐ Window cleaners
☐ Detergents
☐ Nail polish
☐ Gasoline
☐ Wood stove fumes
☐ Garages
☐ Deodorants
☐ Smoke
☐ Pungent foods

HOUSE DUST MITES

Dust mites' excretion and decayed body parts can be a powerful and common trigger of asthma symptoms. These creatures live and feed in soft-surfaced places such as mattresses, couches, pillows and carpets, where there is an abundant supply of naturally shed human skin.

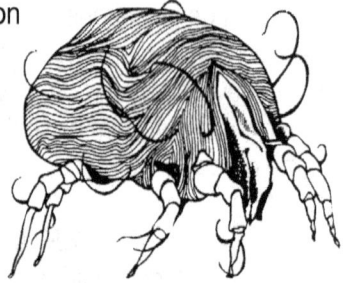

Dust mites proliferate when temperatures are warm and the humidity in the home is high (more than 50%). They cannot survive in dry environments.

Although mites look threatening (although they are too small to see with the naked eye), they do not bite, live on your skin or harm humans, other than creating the triggers for asthma or causing allergies.

PREVENTATIVE MEASURES

☞ Use a dehumidifier to reduce the relative humidity to below 50%.

☞ Keep the house cooler, especially the bedroom. Air conditioning may be necessary in the summer months.

☞ Encase your mattresses, box springs and pillows in allergen-barrier, zippered covers, and wipe the covers frequently.

☞ Launder bed linens in very hot water (55° Celsius).

MOLD

Molds are fungi which can be found just about anywhere where it is damp and/or highly humid and where air flow is minimal–basements, bathrooms and crawl spaces. They also flourish in decaying plant life or on stored foods. As molds grow, they give off spores which become airborne and when inhaled by someone with asthma, can bring on symptoms.

PREVENTATIVE MEASURES

☞ Check all sources of dampness and repair the cause of the dampness.

☞ Install a dehumidifier to ensure less humidity in the home.

☞ Use a fan to improve air circulation in problem areas.

☞ Frequently clean furnace filters, air conditioners, dehumidifiers, vaporizers and other appliances to prevent mold formation.

☞ Damp clothes should be laundered immediately.

☞ Implement general measures for preventing mold such as: using mold-resistant paint for walls; wash window ledges and shower stalls with Lysol or bleach; eliminate or minimize houseplants or cover soil with aluminum foil; use borax or boric acid in wallpaper paste; quick dry shower curtains and towels and avoid clutter.

Be aware of the danger areas for sources of mold such as attics, crawl spaces, bathroom tiles, showers, damp closets, potted plants, refrigerator trays, soil surfaces, old bedding, stored foods and unfinished basements.

PETS

Cats, dogs, gerbils, hamsters, rabbits, mice, rats, guinea pigs, birds and horses can trigger asthma. It is not just the fur or feathers–asthma symptoms can be triggered by the animal's saliva, oil secretions, dander (tiny particles of skin) or urine and feces.

Removal of the pet from the home is the single most effective option for avoiding asthma symptoms from this trigger. There is no such thing as an allergy-free dog or cat. All furred animals shed dander. If you keep your pet you will be increasing the severity of your asthma over time.

PREVENTATIVE MEASURES
(if you keep your pet)

☞ Use a central vacuum system or HEPA vacuum.

☞ Frequently have your air ducts professionally cleaned. Remove carpeting from your home.

☞ Do not allow the pet in the bedroom, on upholstered furniture or other soft surfaces.

☞ Have the pet professionally cleaned or at least by someone else; there are shampoos which can reduce airborne dander.

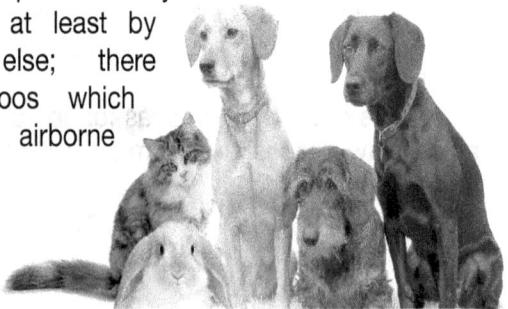

TOBACCO SMOKE

Everyone knows smoking is not healthy. When you have asthma smoking or second-hand exposure to tobacco smoke can bring on asthma symptoms and possibly an asthma attack.

If you have asthma there should be absolutely no smoking within the home, in the car or anywhere else you spend a lot of time.

If you do smoke, it is vital that you become motivated to quit, difficult as it is.

There is now plenty of help to make quitting an easier process. There are medications and nicotine substitutes which your physician can advise you about. Also your pharmacy will have a wide variety of nicotine substitutes that can be purchased without a prescription.

You will probably need to talk to a professional and obtain support from friends and family member to help you through the difficult period of quitting.

Quitting is mostly a psychological issue; most people who successfully quit have tried many times before being successful. Medications and nicotine substitutes can get you through the early difficult times. Equally important is the preparation time, planning to change your lifestyle to accommodate not smoking and setting a quit date that you will commit to.

PREVENTATIVE MEASURES

☞ Visit your physician and ask for help.

☞ Obtain professional counseling on how to quit.

☞ Read all about smoking, visit internet sites, etc. The more information you assimilate, the stronger your motivation will become to quit.

☞ Realistically plan how you have to change your lifestyle and surroundings to minimize the temptation and make it psychologically easier for you to quit.

☞ Establish a quit date that you feel comfortable with.

☞ On the countdown to the quit date start cutting down the number of cigarettes you smoke.

☞ Obtain the necessary medications and/or nicotine substitution products before the quit date and follow the instructions from your pharmacist, physician or nurse.

☞ Quit smoking on the quit day you have planned.

☞ Maintain quitting by celebrating just one day at a time; reward yourself each day and keep to your plan.

If you falter and have a cigarette, don't be hard on yourself. Congratulate yourself for the time you were off cigarettes and start the quitting process over again.

ASTHMA TRIGGERS OUTSIDE

When you're outdoors, you have less control over the triggers you encounter. You cannot, for example, vacuum the lawn if grass pollen is bothering you and there is no air purifier large enough to clean a city's air pollution.

However there are a few things you can do to help reduce your exposure to the outdoor triggers on the following pages.

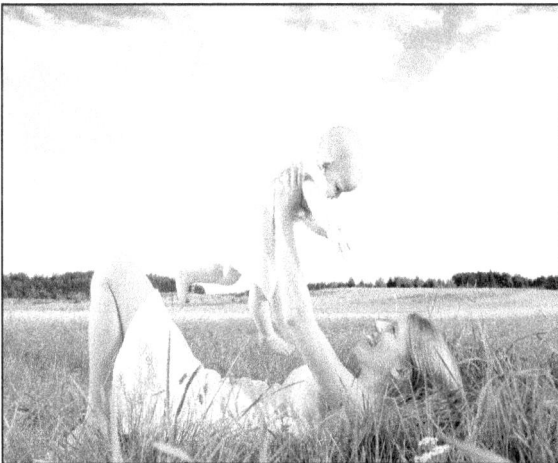

POLLEN

Grass, weed and tree airborne pollens are common triggers for asthma symptoms and are easily inhaled in the warm weather months.

Pollen is the fertilizing agent for plants and different pollens are abundant at different times of the year; millions, sometimes billions of pollens can be released from one plant. A good analogy is to regard them as microscopic balloons, invisible to the naked eye, floating in huge masses over large distances. It helps if you know what type of pollen triggers your asthma. The time of year is a good clue–for example, weeds usually pollinate in the autumn while trees and grasses pollinate in the spring and early summer.

PREVENTATIVE MEASURES

☞ Avoid going outdoors on dry, windy days when pollen counts are high.

☞ Don't plant a lot of trees or shrubs around your house.

☞ Eliminate weeds in your yard and garden.

☞ Check your weather network, newspaper or national allergy bureau for pollen forecasts.

☞ Consider using an air conditioner in the home and car when pollen counts are high.

☞ If you usually exercise outdoors, consider exercising indoors on high pollen count days.

☞ Shower and change your clothing if you have been outside on a high pollen count day.

☞ Consider the use of an air purifier in the home.

☞ Ensure your bedroom is oriented to reducing triggers.

☞ Have your furnace and furnace filter inspected.

☞ Consider regular, professional air duct cleaning.

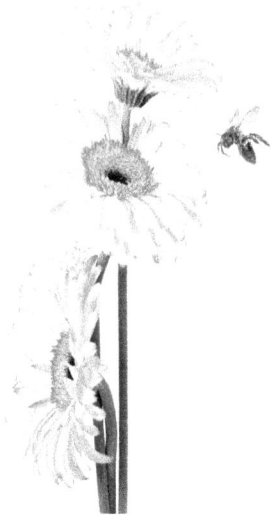

Proper use of medication is the ace in your prevention actions because sometimes you just cannot avoid exposure. Your prescribed or OTC medication will help prevent symptoms. Make sure you are properly instructed in how to use it.

OUTDOOR MOLDS

Outdoor mold, growing on decaying plant life, can be just as problematical as indoor mold. The best preventative measure is to eliminate the source for the mold's growth.

PREVENTATIVE MEASURES

Eliminate the following:

☐ Compost heaps

☐ Grain storage

☐ Piles of leaves

☐ Grass cuttings

☐ Piles of any dead plants

☐ Damp garages

☐ Poorly ventilated spaces like cabins, sheds, cottages

☐ Continuously damp cluttered areas

OUTDOOR AIR POLLUTION

Car fumes, industrial gases, smog, gasoline fumes–the list is endless and there's not much you can do about these pollutants other than trying to avoid them.

PREVENTATIVE MEASURES

☞   Stay indoors on extremely air polluted days.

☞   Make sure the windows in your house are closed.

☞   Use any air cleaning/purifying appliances you have, e.g. air purifier, air conditioner.

☞   Check the weather forecast for smog/pollution warnings.

☞   Wear a mask if you have to go outdoors and you are at risk.

☞   Avoid exercise on high air pollution days.

CLIMATE

Dry, cold air can irritate your airways and trigger asthma symptoms. Sudden changes in the weather can also act as triggers in certain situations.

PREVENTATIVE MEASURES

☞ Warm up through exercises before you go outside.

☞ Wear a scarf around your neck and over your mouth or nose, so that the air is warmed before it reaches your lungs.

☞ Try breathing through your nose to warm up the air before it reaches your lungs.

☞ Dress properly to ensure you keep warm when going outside on a cold day.

☞ Check the weather forecast to ascertain the temperature and see if any sudden changes are expected.

EXERCISE

This trigger can be linked to the climate issue so the two should be considered together. Your physician will tell you that if you are limited in your ability to exercise because of your asthma, it's because your asthma is not being properly controlled. If your asthma is not controlled and you exercise, you may experience worsening symptoms.

Most physicians believe the benefits of regular exercise almost always outweigh the risks associated with exercise-induced asthma.

However, if your asthma is under control and you experience asthma symptoms 5 to 10 minutes after exercising, it could be due to the exercise. This is caused by your airways being sensitive to temperature and humidity changes, especially on a cold day.

The diagnosis of exercise-induced asthma is made by performing a breathing test when you are at rest and then again following exercise. If there is a measured decrease in the speed of the air that can be breathed out following the exercise, it is an indication of exercise-induced asthma.

PREVENTATIVE MEASURES

☞ Consider the measures outlined in climate triggers.

☞ Make sure you are using the right amount of medication prior to exercising (talk to your physician about this).

☞ Make sure air pollution is not a contributing factor.

☞ Plan the right amount of time to exercise in line with the medication you've taken.

☞ High temperatures and the amount of humidity in the air can be a problem.

☞ Always warm up before exercising.

☞ If you develop symptoms while exercising, stop and rest. Take your reliever medication.

☞ Start your exercise slowly. Take your time before attempting more demanding exercise.

☞ Notify teachers or coaches if there is a possibility of exercise triggering asthma symptoms in a school-aged child.

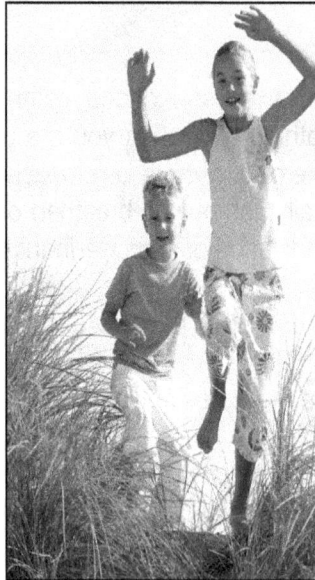

OCCUPATIONAL ASTHMA TRIGGERS

There are a wide variety of fumes, chemicals and other substances which can trigger asthma symptoms in the workplace. Ask yourself the following questions:

• Did your asthma symptoms appear within weeks of starting your current job, or moving to a new area with your job?

• Do your asthma symptoms regularly and predictably occur while at work or within a few hours of leaving the workplace?

• Do you notice your symptoms improve on the weekends or when you are on vacation, and then get worse on returning to work?

• Do other people at work have the same symptoms?

• If you suspect you have occupational asthma, talk to your physician.

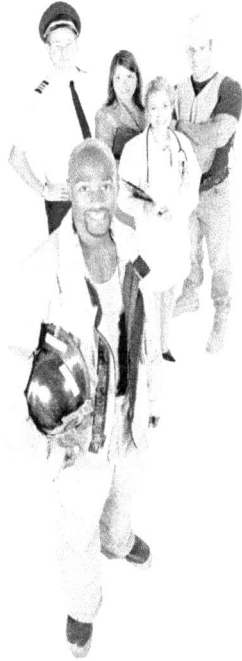

PREVENTATIVE MEASURES

There is no definitive list of risky occupations but here is a list of possible triggers linked to occupations:

☞ **Animals, insects and fungi:** poultry workers, entomologists, laboratory workers and veterinarians.

☞ **Chemicals:** aircraft workers, pulp mill workers, hairdressers, resin manufacturers, dye weighers, brewery workers, electronic workers and refrigeration workers.

☞ **Grains, flours, plants and gums:** bakers, chemists and farmers.

☞ **Isocyanates and metals:** car sprayers, boat builders, foam workers, TDI and refrigerator manufacturers, platinum chemists and refiners, printers, laminators and welders.

☞ **Drugs and enzymes:** Ampicillin, detergent and enzyme manufacturers, pharmacists and pharmaceutical workers.

☞ **Woods:** carpenters, millers, wood finishers, saw mill workers and machinists.

OTHER ASTHMA TRIGGERS

There are a variety of other triggers which can bring on asthma symptoms; the best preventative action is avoidance. The medications, substances and conditions listed below probably lower a person's immunity to asthma symptoms:

Aspirin

Non steroidal anti inflammatories

Sulfites: commonly found in processed potatoes, shrimp, dried fruit, beer and wine

Rhinitis: having a runny or stuffy nose

Sinusitis: having runny or stuffy nasal passages and sinus pain and/or headaches

Allergies: Any sort of allergy can be a precursor to asthma

Colds: You cannot do much against these viral infections, other than adjust your medication as recommended by your physician.

Emotions: Sometimes stress, crying, laughing or extreme emotions can bring on asthma symptoms. Deep breathing or relaxation exercises can sometimes help.

KNOW YOUR ASTHMA TRIGGERS

We have listed a great many triggers; each asthma sufferer has his or her personal triggers. At this stage it is useful to consolidate the list of your triggers and what you intend to do.

My triggers that bring on asthma

....
....
....
....
....
....
....
....
....
....

My preventative actions

....
....
....
....
....
....
....
....
....
....
....
....
....

MONITORING YOUR ASTHMA

The peak flow meter

This small plastic device measures the maximum speed air can be forced out of your lungs. You just take a deep breath and then blow out as hard and as fast as possible. Your physician or respiratory therapist will ask you to blow into it three times and take the highest reading. Many patients have their own peak flow meters; they are quite inexpensive and simple to use. With practice and becoming familiar with your readings it can help in many ways.

What does it tell you?

It tells you how well you are breathing, revealing how open or how narrow your airways are. The peak flow meter can specifically reveal:

If you are about to have an asthma attack (you can then take appropriate preventative action).

Whether your medication is working or not working.

It can help pinpoint actual asthma triggers.

Objectively evaluate how severe an asthma attack you are having.

Is it easy to understand?

First you have to know what your normal peak flow range is–your physician or respiratory therapist can tell you this from your age and height. Then you can see how much lower your reading is from your predicted normal measurement.

When should I take a peak flow measurement?
Early in the morning, in the evening and any time you do not feel well.

How do I read my peak flow measurements?
Your physician will provide you with an action plan linked to how low the readings are compared to your normal reading. A simple and effective way of understanding the seriousness of the readings is to liken the reading to traffic lights.

READING	YOUR RANGE	ACTION REQUIRED
Red Zone	Less than 50%	Follow your emergency action plan, take reliever medication as directed and get to Emergency as quickly as you can.
Yellow Zone High Low	50 - 80% 65 - 80% 50 - 65%	Avoid your asthma triggers, adjust your medication in line with your physician's advice. A low yellow score could be a warning of an imminent asthma attack.
Green Zone	80 – 100%	Maintain your current treatment plan–you are doing well

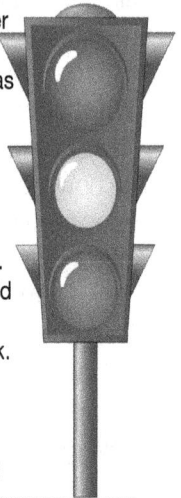

Let's look at a hypothetical case: 12-year-old John is 5'1" tall. Based on his age and height, his physician estimates the normal peak flow meter reading is 361. John visits his aunt who has three cats; on his return home John has trouble breathing and is wheezing. His peak flow rate is 195–he is in the "concern yellow zone" which is 55% of his normal range.

Conclusion

Peak flow meters are the only way you can objectively (numerically) tell how well you are breathing. It provides the green light for You're OK or the red light for Danger, go to Emergency now!

Should you keep a record or diary?

It is difficult to remember precisely what has happened over a period of several weeks so a record or diary of asthma symptoms can be very useful.

Your physician and medical team will decide whether you need a peak flow meter; if you are given one, there will be instructions and maybe a video and/or a diary chart and you will be given your peak flow normal range measurement.

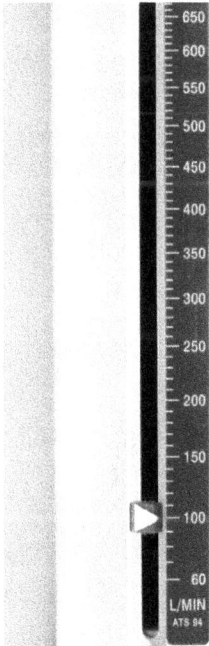

The following pages show an example of a diary sheet with explanations.

Peak Flow Meter Reading

DIARY TO HELP YOU & YOUR PHYSICIAN

The following diary shows peak flow scores, symptoms, medication usage and your comments.

Peak flow scores:

a) Take your "best reading" from three blows and place a 0 for your reading. Join up the 0's and if the line is even, your asthma is controlled. If there are lots of ups and downs this means your asthma is not being controlled

b) Take your reading after using your inhaler. Mark this score with an X so as not to be confused. This line will show how well your medication is working and how well you are breathing.

Symptoms are quantified 0 – 3 levels
Wheeze: 0 None,1 some of exhale, 2 all of exhale, 3 both exhale and inhale
Cough: 0 None, 1 One or less in a minute, 2 one to four in a minute, 3 More than four in a minute.
Sleep: 0 Did not wake, 1 non troubling wheeze or cough, 2 awake two–three times in the night, 3 Awake all night
Nose: 0 None, 1 irritating, 2 runny, 3 very runny
Daily activities: 0 Fully active, 1 restricted running, 2 walking only, 3 missed school / work, stayed inside. If total score 0 you are problem free, 15 is very serious.

Medicines: are recorded
Triggers: try to identify associated causes that brought on an attack e.g. cooking smells, cold weather, emotions etc

This diary can provide many clues and an objective understanding of your asthma condition for your physician and medical team.

Asthma Diary ... Your Asthma Jigsaw Puzzle — SAMPLE

Name: **EMMA**
Please bring to your Doctor's office

PEAK FLOW SCORE

- GREEN ZONE
- CAUTION YELLOW
- CONCERN YELLOW
- DANGER RED

Mark peak flow score with O (before inhaling Bronchodilator) and x (after inhaling Bronchodilator)

Date: JULY 23 2007	SUN		MON		TUE		WED		THUR		FRI		SAT		SUN		MON		TUE		WED		THUR		FRI		SAT	
Time	AM 9	PM 6	AM 6	PM 8	AM 6	PM 8	AM 9	PM 8	AM 8	PM 6	AM 8	PM 5	AM 10	PM 6	AM 9	PM 8	AM 8	PM 8	AM 6	PM 8	AM 7	PM 6	AM 8	PM 6	AM 8	PM 6	AM 10	PM 7

SYMPTOMS

Symptom	SUN	MON	TUE	WED	THUR	FRI	SAT	SUN	MON	TUE	WED	THUR	FRI	SAT
WHEEZE 0-3	1	0	0	0	0	0	0	0	0	0	0	0	0	0
COUGH 0-3	1	1	1	1	0	0	1	1	0	0	0	0	0	0
SLEEP 0-3	0	0	0	0	0	0	1	1	0	1	0	0	0	0
NOSE 0-3	1	0	0	0	0	0	2	1	0	0	0	0	0	0
DAILY ACTIVITIES 0-3														
TOTAL SCORE 0-15	3	1	1	1	0	0	5	3	0	1	0	0	0	0

MEDICINES

Name & Dosage *(tick when taken)*

Medicine	SUN	MON	TUE	WED	THUR	FRI	SAT	SUN	MON	TUE	WED	THUR	FRI	SAT
VENTOLIN .5CC	✓✓	✓✓	✓✓	✓✓	✓✓	✓✓	✓✓	✓	✓✓	✓✓	✓✓	✓✓	✓✓	✓✓
PRELONE 1 1/2 C.	✓✓	✓✓	✓✓	✓✓	✓✓	✓								

COMMENTS

Identified triggers, feelings, medication adjustments, etc. Turn page to write in column.

- I Am Tired
- I Have A Cold
- Getting Better
- Friend Painting
- Stomach Ache

Asthma Diary ... *Your Asthma Jigsaw Puzzle*

Name: _____
Please bring to your Doctor's office

Date
Time

	SUN		MON		TUE		WED		THUR		FRI		SAT		SUN		MON		TUE		WED		THUR		FRI		SAT	
	AM	PM	AM	PM	AM	PM	AM	PM	AM	PM	AM	PM	AM	PM	AM	PM	AM	PM	AM	PM	AM	PM	AM	PM	AM	PM	AM	PM
	9	6	8	6	8	6	9	6	8	6	8	5	10	6	9	6	8	6	8	6	7	6	8	6	8	6	10	7

PEAK FLOW SCORE
Mark peak flow score with O (before inhaling Bronchodilator) and X (after inhaling Bronchodilator)

- GREEN ZONE
- CAUTION YELLOW
- CONCERN YELLOW
- DANGER RED

SYMPTOMS

- WHEEZE 0 - 3
- COUGH 0 - 3
- SLEEP 0 - 3
- NOSE 0 - 3
- DAILY ACTIVITIES 0 - 3
- TOTAL SCORE 0 - 15

MEDICINES

Name & Dosage (tick when taken)

COMMENTS

Identified triggers, feelings, medication adjustments, etc. Turn page to write in column.

MEDICATIONS FOR ASTHMA

This is the domain of your physician but to maintain balance and control of your asthma there are two main types of medications:

Reliever medications (also known as bronchodilators): These medications, as the name implies, give you immediate relief from symptoms. They work by relaxing the tight muscles around the airways, making it easier to breathe. YOU ALWAYS INHALE RELIEVERS.

There are various ways you can inhale and you should make sure you are well trained in the use of your inhalation device. By using the right techniques you will ensure you will get the most out of your inhaled medication.

Always check with your pharmacist and/or physician concerning the right way to use your reliever medication.

Preventer medications: These should be taken on a regular basis even when you are feeling well. They get to the root of the problem–inflammation in the airways.

You should take this medication on a regular basis (it is not used for emergency relief) to ensure long term control and prevent your asthma from getting worse.

Some people forget to take these medications because they do not provide instant relief from symptoms. Your physician will prescribe how often each day you should take them and you can always check with your pharmacist if you have any questions or concerns. It is possible to take more than one preventer medication; again, your physician will decide this.

Conclusion:

It is important to know which medication is the reliever medication in case you are having an asthma attack–do not get the two types (preventer or reliever) confused. The reliever medication is the one you take when having severe symptoms.

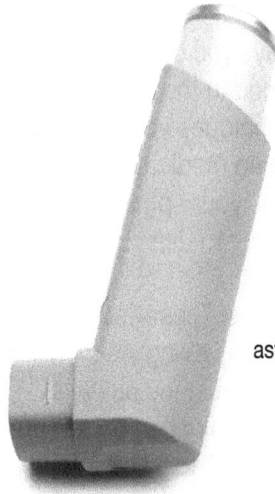

asthma Inhaler

Your Medication Checklist

Name of medicine(s)

....

....

When and how much to take

....

....

How long to take it

....

....

What does the medicine do and when
will you feel it working

....

....

What to do if you forget to take it

....

....

Side effects and what to do about them

....

....

When to call your physician or Emergency

....

....

YOUR EMERGENCY ACTION PLAN

Now that you are familiar with warning signs and peak flow meter readings, you should prepare your own specific action plan. Answer the following questions to help you develop your treatment plan and emergency action plan.

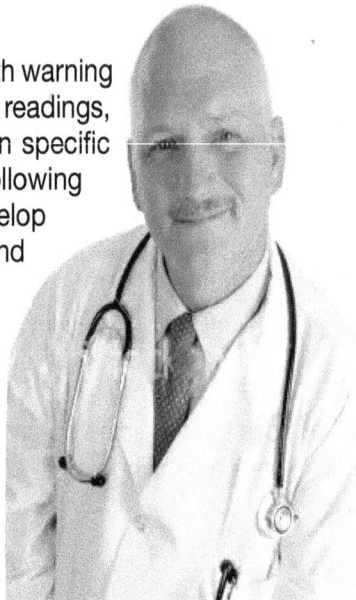

What are your warning signs?

....

....

....

....

What does your physician want you to do when you experience warning signs?

....

....

....

What should you do if your medicines do not seem to be working ?

....

....

Where should you go to get help quickly?

....

....

Should you call your physician or go straight to Emergency?

....

What should you do if you have an asthma emergency late at night?

....

....

When you call your physician, nurse or emergency do you know the following?

Symptoms

....

....

When you took your last medicine

....

....

What actual medicines you have taken

....

....

Your peak flow reading

....

....

USEFUL INFORMATION WEBSITES

All allergy and asthma internet listings*
www.allallergy.net

Allergy Asthma Information Association (AAIA)
www.aaia.ca

Allergy and Asthma Network of Mothers of Asthmatics
www.aanma.org

American Academy of Allergy, Asthma and Immunology (AAAAI)
www.aaaai.org

Allergy Foundation of Canada
www.allergyfoundation.ca

MedicAlert
www.medicalert.com

National Air Duct Cleaners Association (NADCA)
www.nadca.com

Pollen counts
www.pollen.com

* This site enables you to navigate to almost all internet websites regarding asthma, allergy and related topics and resources. This site is highly recommended.

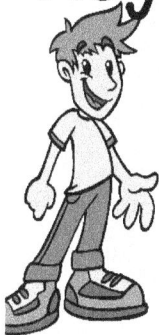

Hey
Babysitter, Nanny,
Caregiver, Teacher or Friend

ASTHMA EMERGENCY ACTION PLAN
In case of a possible Severe Asthma Attack

Place child's photo here

Child's name:	Medic Alert #:
Nickname:	Home phone:
Address:	Cell phone:
Date of Birth:	Work phone:
Parent / guardian:	Emergency phone OR 911
Doctor's name:	Doctor's phone:

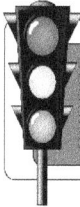

I Have No Asthma Symptoms.

I Have Asthma Symptoms,
But I am in Control.

I Am In Danger and Need Help!

RED ZONE WARNING SYMPTOMS AND SIGNS

- Extreme cough, wheeze or chest tightness.
- Shortness of breath, getting worse.
- Difficulty walking or talking.
- Hard time breathing.
- Hunched over, struggling to breathe.
- Reliever drug is not helping symptoms.
- Peak flow meter reading is less than 50% of personal best.
- Cannot perform usual activities.
- Feeling faint and / or frightened.
- Lips and fingernails are blue.
- The attack came on suddenly.

WHAT TO DO

1. **TELEPHONE 911** for emergency medical help and tell the dispatcher:
"A CHILD IS HAVING A LIFE THREATENING ASTHMA ATTACK."

2. **WHEN IN DOUBT** get to hospital emergency room as efficiently as possible.

OUR CHILD CAN HAVE AN ASTHMA ATTACK IF EXPOSED TO ANY OF THE FOLLOWING:
Tobacco Smoke • Dust Mites • Animals • Cockroaches • Outdoor grass, weed, tree pollen
• Molds • Strong Fumes • Exercise (when asthma not controlled)

☐ Peanuts ☐ Tree nuts ☐ Milk ☐ All dairy ☐ Eggs ☐ Shellfish ☐ Fish

Food additives (list)

Medications (list)

Others

OTHER EMERGENCY CONTACT INFORMATION

Asthma Emergency Action Poster
Available at your local pharmacy
or
email mediscript30@yahoo.ca